This book was compiled by Daniel Melehi
with the A.I assistance of Inventabot

### <u>Dedication</u>
I hope this helps all of my wonderful
readers achieve all their goals in their
business. And I would like to thank my
wonderful wife for all of her continued
support in all my ventures.

©Daniel Melehi

May 7 2023

# Contents

# Chapter 4: Seeing Clearly

Clear vision is something that is essential for performing daily activities such as driving or reading. When our vision is blurry, it can be frustrating and can also hinder our ability to do certain tasks. Fortunately, there are solutions available to help correct vision problems. This chapter will discuss corrective lenses and eye surgery, two common methods used to improve vision.

## SUBCHAPTER 4.1: CORRECTIVE LENSES

Corrective lenses are a popular and effective way to improve vision problems such as refractive errors. Glasses and contact lenses are the two main types of corrective lenses used today. Glasses are made up of lenses that are designed to correct specific refractive errors in the eye. Myopia, hyperopia, and astigmatism can all be corrected with the use of glasses. The lenses in glasses can be made from a variety of materials, including plastic and glass. There are different types of lenses available for different vision needs, such as bifocals for people who need both near and far correction. Contact lenses are thin, curved pieces of plastic that are placed directly on the eye's surface. They are an alternative to glasses and are also used to correct refractive errors. While contacts may be more convenient for people who play sports or have an active lifestyle, they may not be a suitable option for everyone. Proper cleaning and maintenance of contact lenses is crucial in reducing the risk of infection and ensuring that they work effectively.

# SUBCHAPTER 4.2: EYE SURGERY

Eye surgery is another option available to correct vision problems. There are different types of eye surgery available, each targeting different vision problems. Some common types of eye surgery include LASIK and cataract surgery. LASIK, or Laser-Assisted In Situ Keratomileusis, is a type of refractive surgery used to correct myopia, hyperopia, and astigmatism. During the procedure, a laser is used to reshape the cornea, allowing light to enter the eye more accurately. LASIK has become a popular option for people who are looking for a permanent solution to their vision problems. Cataract surgery is a surgical procedure used to remove a cloudy lens from the eye and replace it with an artificial lens. This surgery is typically used to treat cataracts, which is a common age-related condition that causes clouding of the eye's natural lens. After cataract surgery, patients often report improved vision and a reduction in symptoms such as glare and blurry vision. Seeing clearly is important for performing everyday tasks and maintaining overall quality of life. Glasses, contact lenses, and eye surgery are all effective options to correct vision problems and help people see clearly. It is important to talk to an eye doctor about which option is best for individual needs.

# Chapter 1: Understanding the Eye

The eye is one of the most complex organs in the human body. Through it, we are able to perceive the world around us and appreciate its beauty. However, understanding how the eye works can be challenging. In this chapter, we will explore the anatomy of the eye and how it functions.

# SUBCHAPTER 1.1: ANATOMY OF THE EYE

The eye is made up of several structures that work together to transmit visual information to the brain. These structures include the cornea, iris, lens, retina, optic nerve, and vitreous. The cornea is the clear, outermost part of the eye that covers the iris and pupil. It helps to refract light and protect the eye from foreign objects. The iris is the colored part of the eye that controls the amount of light that enters the eye by adjusting the size of the pupil. The lens is located behind the iris and focuses light onto the retina. The retina is a layer of tissue that lines the back of the eye and contains photoreceptor cells that help to convert light into electrical signals that are transmitted to the brain. The optic nerve is a bundle of nerve fibers that carries these electrical signals to the brain. The vitreous is a gel-like substance that fills the space between the retina and the lens.

# SUBCHAPTER 1.2: HOW THE EYE WORKS

The process of vision begins when light enters the eye through the cornea. The cornea refracts the light and focuses it onto the lens. The lens then adjusts its shape to focus the light onto the retina. The photoreceptor cells in the retina then convert the light into electrical signals that are transmitted along the optic nerve to the brain. Once the electrical signals reach the brain, they are processed and interpreted, allowing us to see and make sense of the world around us. This complex process happens in a fraction of a second and is essential for our survival and well-being. In the next chapter, we will discuss some of the most common eye disorders, including refractive errors, cataracts, glaucoma, age-related macular degeneration, and diabetic retinopathy.

# SUBCHAPTER 1.1: ANATOMY OF THE EYE

The eye is one of the most complex and fascinating organs in the human body. It is responsible for receiving and processing light and turning it into the images that we see. To understand how the eye works, it is essential to understand its anatomy. The eye is made up of several parts, including the cornea, iris, pupil, lens, retina, and optic nerve. The cornea is the transparent outermost layer that covers the front of the eye. It is responsible for focusing the light that enters the eye, much like a camera lens. The iris is the colored part of the eye that surrounds the pupil. Its function is to regulate the amount of light that enters the eye. The pupil is the black circular opening in the center of the iris that allows light to enter the eye. The lens is a crystal-clear structure located behind the iris and the pupil. Its function is to focus the light onto the retina. The retina is a thin layer of tissue that lines the back of the eye. It contains millions of light-sensitive cells called rods and cones that convert the light into electrical signals that are sent to the brain via the optic nerve. The optic nerve is a bundle of nerve fibers that carries the electrical signals from the retina to the brain, where they are interpreted as images. In addition to these structures, the eye also contains several other important components, such as the sclera, the choroid, and the vitreous humor. The sclera is the white, outer covering of the eye, while the choroid is a layer of blood vessels that supplies nutrients to the retina. The vitreous humor is a jelly-like substance that fills the space between the lens and the retina. Understanding the anatomy of the eye is essential for understanding how it works and for diagnosing and treating various eye disorders that can affect vision.

# SUBCHAPTER 1.2: HOW THE EYE WORKS

The human eye is a complex organ, responsible for one of our most important senses: vision. It works by detecting and processing light through a series of structures that work together in a coordinated and efficient manner. The process starts with light entering the eye through the cornea, a clear outer covering that refracts or bends the light. The light then travels through the pupil, a circular opening in the center of the iris, which is the colored part of the eye. The iris controls the size of the pupil to regulate the amount of light that enters the eye. The light then passes through the lens, a flexible and clear structure that changes shape to fine-tune the focus of the light onto the retina. The retina is a thin layer of tissue lining the back of the eye and contains millions of specialized light-sensitive cells called photoreceptors that convert light into electrical signals.

Two main types of photoreceptors exist in the retina: rods and cones. Rods are highly sensitive to light and help us see dimly lit objects, while cones are responsible for color vision and detecting fine details. The electrical signals from the photoreceptors are then transmitted to the brain through the optic nerve, which is responsible for transmitting visual information from the eye to the brain. The brain then processes this information to give us the perception of sight. Overall, the eye works like a complex camera with a series of structures working in harmony to ensure we can see the world around us. It's truly remarkable how the eye processes light and translates it into the images we see.

# Chapter 2: Common Eye Disorders

The eyes are one of the most delicate and intricate organs in the body, making them vulnerable to various disorders. In this chapter, we will explore some of the most common eye disorders that affect people worldwide.

## SUBCHAPTER 2.1: REFRACTIVE ERRORS

Refractive errors are the most common type of eye disorders that affect people of all ages. These disorders occur when the shape of the eye prevents light from focusing on the retina, leading to blurred vision. The most common types of refractive errors include:

## Subchapter 2.1.1: Myopia

Myopia, also known as nearsightedness, is a type of refractive error that affects individuals who have difficulty seeing distant objects clearly. This occurs when the eye is too long or the cornea is too curved, causing light to focus in front of the retina. Myopia can be corrected with the use of glasses, contact lenses, or refractive surgery.

## Subchapter 2.1.2: Hyperopia

Hyperopia, also known as farsightedness, is a type of refractive error that affects individuals who have difficulty seeing nearby objects clearly. This occurs when the eye is too short or the cornea is too flat, causing light to focus behind the retina. Hyperopia can also be corrected with the use of glasses, contact lenses, or refractive surgery.

## Subchapter 2.1.3: Astigmatism

Astigmatism is a type of refractive error that occurs when the cornea is irregularly shaped, causing the eye to focus light in more than one place on the retina. This leads to blurred or distorted vision. Astigmatism can be corrected with glasses, contact lenses, or refractive surgery.

## SUBCHAPTER 2.2: CATARACTS

Cataracts are a common eye disorder that occurs when the lens of the eye becomes cloudy, leading to decreased vision and potentially blindness. Cataracts are typically age-related, but can also be caused by injury, certain medications, or other underlying health conditions. Treatment for cataracts typically involves surgery to remove the cloudy lens and replace it with an artificial lens implant.

## SUBCHAPTER 2.3: GLAUCOMA

Glaucoma is a group of eye disorders that cause damage to the optic nerve, typically due to high pressure inside the eye. If left untreated, glaucoma can lead to vision loss and eventually blindness. Treatment for glaucoma typically involves the use of eye drops to reduce intraocular pressure, or surgery in more severe cases.

# SUBCHAPTER 2.4: AGE-RELATED MACULAR DEGENERATION

Age-related macular degeneration (AMD) is a common eye disorder that affects individuals over the age of 50, causing damage to the macula of the eye and leading to central vision loss. AMD is typically categorized as either dry or wet, with the dry form being more common and less severe. Treatment for AMD typically involves the use of vitamins and supplements, lifestyle changes, and in some cases, injections or laser surgery.

# SUBCHAPTER 2.5: DIABETIC RETINOPATHY

Diabetic retinopathy is a common eye disorder that affects individuals who have diabetes, causing damage to the blood vessels in the retina and leading to vision loss. Treatment for diabetic retinopathy typically involves blood sugar control, lifestyle changes, and in severe cases, laser surgery or injections. In conclusion, understanding the common eye disorders is essential in maintaining proper eye health. With early detection and treatment, many of these conditions can be managed effectively, allowing individuals to maintain their vision and overall quality of life.

## SUBCHAPTER 2.1: REFRACTIVE ERRORS

Refractive errors are the most common type of eye disorders, affecting both children and adults. These errors occur when the shape of the eye prevents light from focusing directly on the retina.

## Myopia

Myopia, also known as nearsightedness, is a refractive error where distant objects appear blurry while nearby objects are clear. This occurs when the eyeball is too long or the cornea is too curved, causing light to focus in front of the retina instead of on it. Myopia can be corrected with glasses, contact lenses, or refractive surgery.

# Hyperopia

Hyperopia, also known as farsightedness, is a refractive error where nearby objects appear blurry while distant objects are clear. This occurs when the eyeball is too short or the cornea is too flat, causing light to focus behind the retina instead of on it. Hyperopia can be corrected with glasses, contact lenses, or refractive surgery.

# Astigmatism

Astigmatism is a refractive error where the front of the eye is irregularly shaped, causing light to focus at multiple points instead of just one. This can result in blurry or distorted vision at any distance. Astigmatism can be corrected with glasses, contact lenses, or refractive surgery. It is important to have regular eye exams to detect and diagnose any refractive errors, as they can lead to eye strain, fatigue, and headaches if left untreated. Treatment options can greatly improve vision and overall quality of life for those with refractive errors.

## SUBCHAPTER 2.1.1: MYOPIA

Myopia, commonly known as nearsightedness, is a common eye disorder that affects a significant percentage of the population. People with myopia can see near objects clearly but struggle to see objects in the distance. This condition occurs when the eyeball is too long or the cornea is too curved. As a result, the light that enters the eye is focused in the front of the retina instead of on the retina, causing distant objects to appear blurry. Myopia can develop in childhood or adolescence and can progressively worsen until the mid-20s. However, in some cases, it can progress throughout adulthood. Symptoms of myopia include squinting, eye strain, headaches, and difficulty seeing distant objects such as street signs or a movie screen. Corrective lenses, such as glasses or contact lenses, are commonly prescribed to treat myopia. In some cases, refractive surgery can also be an option. Preventative measures to help reduce the development or worsening of myopia include practicing good eye hygiene, spending time outdoors, taking regular breaks when doing close-up work, and getting regular eye exams. In conclusion, myopia is a common eye disorder that can cause difficulty in seeing distant objects. However, with proper treatment and preventative measures, it is manageable. Consult with an optometrist or ophthalmologist if you or someone you know is experiencing symptoms of myopia.

## SUBCHAPTER 2.1.2: HYPEROPIA

Hyperopia, commonly known as farsightedness, is a condition where distant objects are seen clearly but nearby objects appear blurry. Individuals with hyperopia have an eye that is too short or a cornea that is too flat, causing light entering the eye to focus behind the retina instead of on it. Individuals with mild hyperopia may not experience any symptoms, but those with moderate to severe cases may experience eyestrain, headaches, and have difficulty reading or doing close-up work. Hyperopia can be diagnosed through a comprehensive eye exam that measures the eye's focusing ability and looks for signs of other eye conditions. There are several treatment options for hyperopia, including corrective lenses, such as glasses or contact lenses, or refractive surgery, such as LASIK. Eyeglasses and contact lenses work by bending light to compensate for the shape of the eye, while refractive surgery reshapes the cornea to focus light directly on the retina. It is important to note that with age, the focusing ability of the eye decreases, resulting in difficulty seeing nearby objects, even for individuals without hyperopia. Therefore, regular eye exams are essential in maintaining good overall eye health and detecting any changes in vision. In addition to corrective measures, there are also lifestyle changes that can aid in reducing eyestrain and enhancing the overall health of the eyes. These include taking frequent breaks when working on close-up tasks, positioning the computer screen at an appropriate distance, maintaining a healthy diet rich in vitamins and minerals, and limiting screen time.

## SUBCHAPTER 2.1.3: ASTIGMATISM

Astigmatism is a common eye disorder that affects the way light enters the eye, causing blurred or distorted vision. Unlike nearsightedness or farsightedness, which are caused by an irregular shape of the eyeball, astigmatism occurs when the cornea or lens of the eye has an irregular shape. Symptoms of astigmatism may include headaches, eye strain, and difficulty seeing fine details or reading. Diagnosis of astigmatism is typically done during a routine eye exam, using techniques such as a visual acuity test or a keratometry test. Treatment options for astigmatism vary depending on the severity of the condition. For mild cases, treatment with corrective lenses such as glasses or contacts may be effective in correcting the problem. For more severe cases or for those who do not wish to wear glasses or contacts, refractive surgery may be an option. LASIK and PRK are two common refractive surgeries that can help correct astigmatism by reshaping the cornea. It is important to note that astigmatism can occur in combination with other vision problems, including nearsightedness and farsightedness. If you experience any vision problems, it is important to schedule regular eye exams with your optometrist or ophthalmologist to ensure your eyes are healthy and functioning properly.

# SUBCHAPTER 2.2: CATARACTS

Cataracts occur when the lens of the eye becomes cloudy, causing vision to become blurry or dim. They are a common eye disorder, especially among older adults. There are different types of cataracts, including age-related cataracts, congenital cataracts, and secondary cataracts that can develop as a result of another medical condition, such as diabetes. Symptoms of cataracts include cloudy or blurred vision, sensitivity to glare, difficulty seeing at night, and seeing faded or dull colors. Cataracts can also make it difficult to read or to see clearly when driving. The good news is that cataracts can usually be treated with surgery. During cataract surgery, the cloudy lens is removed and replaced with an artificial lens. It's important to get regular eye exams to monitor cataract development, especially if you are over 50 years old or have risk factors such as diabetes or a family history of cataracts. In addition, wearing sunglasses and a hat with a wide brim to protect your eyes from the sun can help prevent cataracts from forming. Quitting smoking and maintaining a healthy diet can also reduce your risk of developing cataracts. If you have cataracts, don't worry - modern cataract surgery is safe and effective, and can restore your vision to its former clarity. Talk to your eye doctor if you have any concerns about cataracts or any other eye disorders.

# SUBCHAPTER 2.3: GLAUCOMA

Glaucoma is a group of eye conditions that damage the optic nerve, which is responsible for transmitting visual information from the eye to the brain. This damage is often caused by high pressure inside the eye, known as intraocular pressure. There are several types of glaucoma, but the most common type is called primary open-angle glaucoma. This type of glaucoma develops slowly and can cause irreversible vision loss if left untreated. It often has no symptoms until significant visual damage has occurred. In addition to intraocular pressure, other factors such as age, family history, and certain medical conditions may increase the risk of developing glaucoma. Regular eye exams and early detection of glaucoma are important to prevent vision loss. Treatment for glaucoma often involves lowering intraocular pressure through eye drops, oral medications, laser therapy or surgery. Follow-up eye exams and monitoring are important to ensure the effectiveness of treatment and prevent further vision loss. If you have a family history of glaucoma or are experiencing symptoms such as blurred vision, halos around lights, or eye pain, it is important to schedule an appointment with an eye doctor as soon as possible. Detecting and treating glaucoma early can help preserve your vision and overall eye health.

# SUBCHAPTER 2.4: AGE-RELATED MACULAR DEGENERATION

Age-related macular degeneration (AMD) is a common eye disorder that affects the macula, the central part of the retina responsible for sharp, clear vision. This condition causes progressive damage to the macular cells, leading to blurriness and distortion of the central vision necessary for reading, driving, and recognizing faces. AMD typically affects people over the age of 50 and is a leading cause of vision loss in older adults. AMD has two types: dry and wet. Dry AMD is the more common form, affecting around 80% of those with the condition. It occurs when the light-sensitive cells in the macula gradually break down, causing a slow loss of central vision. On the other hand, wet AMD is rarer but more severe and aggressive. It occurs when abnormal blood vessels grow beneath the retina and leak blood and fluid, leading to rapid and severe central vision loss if left untreated. Several risk factors increase the likelihood of developing AMD, including age, genetics, smoking, obesity, high blood pressure, and poor nutrition. Although the advanced stage of AMD cannot be cured, treatment and lifestyle changes can slow down the progression and help protect the remaining vision. Treatment for dry AMD may involve taking nutritional supplements with high doses of vitamins C and E, zinc, copper, and lutein to slow the progression of the disease. In some cases, low vision aids like magnifying lenses and special glasses can help improve vision. For wet AMD, the aim of treatment is to stop the growth of abnormal blood vessels in the retina. This can be achieved by injecting anti-VEGF drugs into the eye to reduce inflammation and prevent the growth of new blood vessels. In severe cases, laser surgery may be required to destroy the abnormal blood vessels and prevent further leakage. To reduce the risk of developing AMD, it is important to maintain a healthy lifestyle by avoiding smoking, controlling blood pressure and cholesterol levels, managing weight, and eating a balanced, nutrient-rich diet that includes plenty of leafy greens, fish, and whole grains. Routine eye exams and vision screenings are also crucial for early detection and treatment of AMD. In conclusion, AMD is a serious eye condition that affects millions of people worldwide, particularly those above 50 years old. Being proactive about one's eye health, making lifestyle changes, and undergoing timely treatment can help protect and preserve one's central vision and quality of life.

## SUBCHAPTER 2.5: DIABETIC RETINOPATHY

Diabetic retinopathy is a complication of diabetes and a leading cause of blindness in adults. It occurs when high blood sugar levels cause damage to the blood vessels in the retina, the light-sensitive tissue at the back of the eye. There are two types of diabetic retinopathy: non-proliferative and proliferative. Non-proliferative diabetic retinopathy is the early stage of the disease, where blood vessels in the retina become damaged and begin to leak fluid or blood. This can cause the retina to swell, leading to blurred vision. Proliferative diabetic retinopathy is more severe and occurs when new, abnormal blood vessels begin to grow in the retina. These new blood vessels can lead to further damage and vision loss. Symptoms of diabetic retinopathy include blurry or distorted vision, floaters, dark spots, and difficulty seeing at night. If left untreated, diabetic retinopathy can lead to blindness. The best way to prevent diabetic retinopathy is to control your blood sugar levels through diet, exercise, and medication if necessary. It's also important to have regular eye exams, especially if you have diabetes. Your eye doctor can detect early signs of diabetic retinopathy and provide treatment before it causes permanent vision loss. Treatment for diabetic retinopathy depends on the severity of the disease. In non-proliferative diabetic retinopathy, close monitoring and control of blood sugar levels may be sufficient. In more severe cases, treatment may include laser therapy to help seal leaking blood vessels or injections of medication to stop the growth of abnormal blood vessels. In advanced cases, surgery may be necessary. If you have diabetes, it's important to prioritize your eye health and have regular eye exams. By controlling your blood sugar levels and staying vigilant about your eye health, you can reduce your risk of developing diabetic retinopathy and other eye disorders.

# Chapter 3: Less Common Eye Disorders

The human eye is an incredibly complex organ that can experience a wide variety of disorders. While some conditions like myopia and astigmatism are quite common, others are much less prevalent. This chapter covers some of the less common eye disorders that people may encounter.

# SUBCHAPTER 3.1: RETINAL DETACHMENT

Retinal detachment is a serious condition that occurs when the retina becomes separated from the underlying layers of tissue that support it. This can lead to significant vision loss and even permanent blindness if not treated quickly. There are several risk factors that can increase a person's chances of experiencing retinal detachment. These include previous eye surgery, severe nearsightedness, a history of eye injury, and advancing age. Symptoms of the condition include flashes of light, floaters, and a shadow or curtain that appears to be moving across the field of vision. If you suspect that you may be experiencing retinal detachment, it is essential to seek medical attention right away. Treatment typically involves surgery to reattach the retina to the underlying tissues.

# SUBCHAPTER 3.2:
# KERATOCONUS

Keratoconus is a condition that occurs when the cornea, which is the clear dome-shaped structure that covers the front of the eye, becomes thin and bulges outwards. This can cause significant vision problems, including blurred vision, double vision, and halos around lights. The cause of keratoconus is not entirely understood, but researchers believe that it may be related to a combination of genetic and environmental factors. Treatment for the condition typically depends on how severe it is. In milder cases, eyeglasses or contact lenses may be sufficient to correct vision. However, in more severe cases, surgery may be required to replace the damaged cornea.

# SUBCHAPTER 3.3: COLOR BLINDNESS

Color blindness is a condition in which a person is unable to distinguish between certain colors or perceive colors at all. This can be caused by a variety of genetic factors, and affects both males and females. There are several types of color blindness, including red-green color blindness and blue-yellow color blindness. While there is no cure for the condition, there are certain tools and techniques that can be used to help color blind individuals navigate their surroundings. For example, some people may use special glasses or electronic devices to help them distinguish between different colors.

# SUBCHAPTER 3.4: OPTIC NEUROPATHY

Optic neuropathy is a condition that occurs when the optic nerve, which is responsible for transmitting visual information from the eye to the brain, becomes damaged. This can lead to vision loss, including blind spots and problems with color perception. There are several factors that can increase a person's risk of developing optic neuropathy, including high blood pressure, diabetes, and certain medications. Treatment for the condition typically involves addressing any underlying health conditions and taking steps to preserve the remaining vision. In some cases, surgery may be necessary to repair the damaged optic nerve.

## SUBCHAPTER 3.1: RETINAL DETACHMENT

Retinal detachment occurs when the retina, which is the light-sensitive tissue lining the back of the eye, pulls away from its normal position. This can lead to a loss of vision and must be treated immediately to prevent further damage. Retinal detachment occurs more frequently in people over the age of

50, those who have had previous eye surgery, and those with a family history of the condition. It can be caused by a variety of factors, including trauma to the eye, diabetes, or a vitreous gel that has pulled away from the retina. Symptoms of retinal detachment include sudden onset of floaters or flashes of light, a curtain-like shadow or blurred vision in the peripheral (side) vision. If you experience any of these symptoms, you should see an eye doctor immediately to prevent permanent vision loss. Treatment for retinal detachment involves repairing the retina to its original position. This is typically done through surgery, which may involve laser therapy, cryopexy (freezing), or scleral buckling (placing a band around the eye to push the retina back into place). In more severe cases, a vitrectomy may be necessary to remove the vitreous gel and repair the retina. In summary, retinal detachment is a serious condition that requires prompt medical attention. Symptoms may include floaters, flashes of light, and blurred vision. Treatment options include surgery, laser therapy, cryopexy, and scleral buckling. If you experience any symptoms of retinal detachment, seek medical attention immediately to prevent permanent vision loss.

## SUBCHAPTER 3.2:
## KERATOCONUS

Keratoconus is a progressive eye disease that affects the cornea, the clear window at the front of the eye. The cornea is responsible for focusing light onto the retina. In healthy eyes, the cornea is dome-shaped, but in eyes with keratoconus, the cornea gradually thins and becomes cone-shaped, which distorts vision and causes nearsightedness, irregular astigmatism, and light sensitivity. The exact cause of keratoconus is not known, but it is believed to be partly genetic and also associated with environmental factors such as frequent eye rubbing, chronic eye irritation, and poorly fitted contact lenses. It usually affects both eyes, but one eye may be more severe than the other. Symptoms of keratoconus include blurred and distorted vision, difficulty seeing at night, sensitivity to bright lights and glare, and frequent changes in eyeglass or contact lens prescription. In some cases, keratoconus can progress to the point where a corneal transplant may be necessary to restore vision. Diagnosis of keratoconus involves a comprehensive eye exam, including corneal mapping and analysis of corneal thickness and shape. In some cases, a special imaging test called corneal topography may be used for more detailed analysis. Treatment for keratoconus depends on the severity of the disease. In mild cases, eyeglasses or contact lenses may be sufficient to correct vision. In moderate to severe cases, specialized contact lenses such as scleral lenses or hybrid lenses may be necessary. These lenses are designed to fit the irregularly shaped cornea and provide clearer vision than traditional contact lenses. In advanced cases, corneal cross-linking may be recommended to help strengthen the weakened cornea. During this procedure, eye drops containing a photosensitizing agent are applied to the cornea, followed by exposure to UV light. This helps to strengthen the cornea by creating new cross-links between collagen fibers. In severe cases, a corneal transplant may be necessary to replace the damaged cornea with a healthy donor cornea. This is a major surgery with potential risks and complications, but it can restore vision in many cases. Early detection and treatment of keratoconus is crucial to prevent progression of the disease and preserve vision. Regular eye exams are important for anyone with a family history of keratoconus or symptoms of blurry vision or light sensitivity.

## SUBCHAPTER 3.3: COLOR BLINDNESS

Color blindness, also known as color vision deficiency, is a genetic condition that affects the ability to distinguish between colors. People with this condition have difficulty seeing certain colors or distinguishing between them.

## Causes of Color Blindness

Color blindness is caused by a genetic mutation that affects the development of the cone cells in the retina. There are three types of cone cells, each of which is responsible for detecting a different color: green, red, and blue. In people with color blindness, one or more of these cone types do not function properly, leading to difficulty in distinguishing between certain colors.

## Symptoms of Color Blindness

The symptoms of color blindness vary depending on the severity of the condition. Some people may have difficulty distinguishing between certain shades of red and green, while others may not be able to see any colors at all. In severe cases, people may see the world in shades of gray.

# Treatment for Color Blindness

Currently, there is no cure for color blindness. However, there are several tools and techniques available to help those who have difficulty seeing certain colors. One common tool is the use of color correction glasses, which help to filter out specific wavelengths of light to enhance color vision. Another technique is the use of computer programs and smartphone apps that can adjust color settings to make them more distinguishable for people with color blindness.

# Living with Color Blindness

While color blindness can be frustrating and create challenges, it is a manageable condition. Those who are diagnosed with color blindness can still lead normal, healthy lives and pursue any career they desire. It is important to note that individuals with color blindness may need to seek accommodations in certain settings, such as taking color-coded tests or working with certain types of electronics that rely on color-coding. In these situations, it is best to be open and communicative with instructors and employers to find solutions that work for everyone.

# Conclusion

Color blindness is a condition that affects a significant percentage of the population. While it may create challenges, it is important to remember that it is a manageable condition. By understanding the causes and symptoms of color blindness, individuals can seek out the necessary tools and accommodations to lead a normal, healthy life.

## SUBCHAPTER 3.4: OPTIC NEUROPATHY

Optic neuropathy refers to damage to the optic nerve that transmits visual information from the eyes to the brain. This can occur due to a variety of reasons, such as injury, inflammation, and diseases like glaucoma and multiple sclerosis. One common type of optic neuropathy is ischemic optic neuropathy. This occurs when there is insufficient blood flow to the optic nerve, leading to damage and loss of vision. Ischemic optic neuropathy is more common in older adults and those with conditions like diabetes and high blood pressure. Another type of optic neuropathy is compressive optic neuropathy, which occurs when there is pressure on the optic nerve. This can be caused by conditions like a brain tumor, an aneurysm, or an enlarged thyroid gland. Symptoms of optic neuropathy can vary depending on its cause and severity. Common symptoms include: - Decreased vision - Blurred vision - Loss of peripheral vision - Color vision changes - Pain in the eye - Headache Treatment for optic neuropathy depends on the underlying cause. In some cases, such as with ischemic optic neuropathy, little can be done to restore lost vision. However, there are treatment options that can help slow down or prevent further damage to the optic nerve. These may include medications, eye drops, or even surgery in some cases. It's important to have regular eye exams and to seek medical attention if you experience any changes in your vision. Early detection and treatment of optic neuropathy can help prevent further damage and potentially even restore some lost vision.

# Chapter 4: Seeing Clearly

Achieving and maintaining clear vision is important for a healthy and productive life. In this chapter, we'll discuss the different methods used to correct vision problems, including corrective lenses and eye surgery.

## SUBCHAPTER 4.1: CORRECTIVE LENSES

Corrective lenses, including glasses and contact lenses, are the most common method of correcting refractive errors, such as myopia, hyperopia, and astigmatism.

Glasses work by bending light rays that enter the eye and positioning them to correctly focus on the retina. Contact lenses work in a similar way, but they sit directly on the eye's surface instead of on frames in front of your eyes. There are several different types of lenses available, including single vision lenses, bifocal lenses, and progressive lenses. Single vision lenses have the same power throughout the lens and are used to correct a single vision problem such as myopia or hyperopia. Bifocal lenses contain two prescriptions in one lens and are used to correct both near and far vision problems. Progressive lenses, also called no-line bifocals, provide a gradual change in prescription over the lens and are used to correct presbyopia, a condition that causes difficulty seeing up close as we age. It is important to have a comprehensive eye exam regularly to ensure that your corrective lenses are still appropriate for your vision needs.

# SUBCHAPTER 4.2: EYE SURGERY

For some people, corrective lenses may not be enough to correct their vision problems. Eye surgery, also known as refractive surgery, can be considered to permanently reshape the cornea, the clear front surface of the eye, to improve the focusing power of the eye. There are several types of refractive surgery, including LASIK, PRK, and LASEK. The most common is LASIK, which uses a laser to reshape the cornea under a thin flap of tissue. PRK and LASEK use a laser to reshape the cornea without creating a flap of tissue. While eye surgery can be effective in correcting refractive errors, it is important to remember that it is still a surgical procedure and carries risks. It is important to discuss the risks and benefits with your eye doctor and ensure that you are a good candidate for the procedure.

# Conclusion

Correcting vision problems is crucial for maintaining a high quality of life. Fortunately, there are several methods available to effectively correct vision problems, including corrective lenses and eye surgery. Consult with your eye doctor to determine which method is best for you and remember to have regular eye exams to ensure that your vision remains clear.

## SUBCHAPTER 4.1: CORRECTIVE LENSES

Corrective lenses are a common solution for people who suffer from refractive errors, such as myopia, hyperopia, and astigmatism. These are eyeglasses or contact lenses that are prescribed by an eye doctor to improve vision by refracting light that enters the eye. There are different types of corrective lenses available, depending on the individual's needs and preferences. Eyeglasses are the most common type of corrective lens. They consist of a frame that supports two lenses, each with a specific prescription. The lenses can be made of glass, plastic, or polycarbonate and can be tinted to protect the eyes from the sun's harmful UV rays. Contact lenses are another popular option for people who don't want to wear eyeglasses. They are small, thin lenses that are placed directly on the eye's surface. Contact lenses can be made of soft or rigid materials and can be used for a range of refractive errors. There are also specialized types of corrective lenses available, such as bifocals, trifocals, and progressive lenses. Bifocals have two segments on each lens, with the top for distance vision and the bottom for near vision. Trifocals have three segments on each lens, with the top for distance vision, the middle for intermediate vision, and the bottom for near vision. Progressive lenses have a gradual change in lens power from the top to the bottom, providing clear vision at all distances. It's essential to have a regular eye exam to check if your corrective lenses need to be updated. Wearing outdated lenses can cause eye strain, headaches, and other problems. Also, make sure to follow the care instructions for your corrective lenses to ensure they last longer and provide optimal vision. In conclusion, corrective lenses are an effective solution for many people who suffer from refractive errors. Whether you prefer eyeglasses or contact lenses, there are different types of lenses available to suit your needs and preferences. It's important to have regular eye exams and follow the care instructions for your lenses to ensure that they are providing optimal vision.

## EYE SURGERY

Eye surgery is an advanced medical procedure used to correct eye problems that cannot be addressed using corrective lenses. There are several types of eye surgery, but all of them aim to improve vision in the affected eye. One common type of eye surgery is *LASIK* (Laser-Assisted in Situ Keratomileusis). This procedure involves using a laser to reshape the cornea, which is the clear, dome-shaped surface that covers the front of the eye. LASIK surgery can correct nearsightedness, farsightedness and astigmatism. Recovery time is typically quick, and most patients experience a noticeable improvement in vision within a couple of days. Another type of eye surgery is *cataract surgery*. Cataracts occur when the lens of the eye becomes cloudy, causing vision to become blurry or hazy. During cataract surgery, the cloudy lens is removed and replaced with a clear artificial lens. This procedure is safe and highly effective, and can greatly improve a patient's visual clarity. For patients with age-related macular degeneration (AMD), which is a common cause of vision loss in older adults, there are several surgical options available. One of these is the *macular translocation surgery*. This procedure involves moving the macula, which is the part of the retina responsible for fine central vision, to a healthier part of the eye. Another option is *anti-angiogenesis therapy,* where medication is injected into the eye to prevent abnormal blood vessels from forming. Other types of eye surgery include *glaucoma surgery*, which can help lower intraocular pressure and prevent damage to the optic nerve. There is also *corneal transplant surgery*, where a damaged or diseased cornea is replaced with a healthy donor cornea. While eye surgery can be highly effective in treating many eye conditions, it is important to note that all surgeries carry some degree of risk. Patients should discuss the risks and benefits of any eye surgery with their eye doctor before undergoing the procedure.

## Conclusion

Eye surgery can be a highly effective way to address many types of eye problems that cannot be corrected with corrective lenses. LASIK, cataract surgery, and macular translocation surgery are just some of the surgical options available to patients. However, it is important for patients to understand that all surgeries carry some degree of risk, and they should discuss these risks with their eye doctor before undergoing any procedure.

# Chapter 5: Preventing Eye Disorders

The eyes are windows to the world, and it is important to take care of them throughout life. Although some eye disorders may be unavoidable, there are still many ways to prevent them or minimize their impact. In this chapter, we will discuss some techniques and habits that can be incorporated into everyday life to maintain eye health.

## SUBCHAPTER 5.1: HEALTHY LIFESTYLE HABITS

A balanced and healthy lifestyle is pivotal to maintaining good eye health. It is essential to consume a diet rich in vitamins and minerals that are particularly beneficial for the eyes. Vitamins such as A, C, and E, as well as minerals such as zinc and copper, are essential for good ocular health. A diet high in fruits, vegetables, and fish can supply these nutrients. Regular physical activity is also linked to decreased risk of eye disorders, such as age-related macular degeneration and glaucoma. Exercise increases blood flow to the eyes and reduces intraocular pressure, both of which are vital to the well-being of the eyes. Protecting the eyes from harmful ultraviolet (UV) rays is another crucial aspect of maintaining good eye health. Too much UV exposure can accelerate the development of cataracts and other eye disorders. Wearing sunglasses that block at least 99% of harmful UV rays when outdoors can minimize the risk.

## SUBCHAPTER 5.2: EYE EXAMS AND SCREENINGS

Preventive eye care involves ensuring regular eye exams and screenings. Many eye disorders, such as glaucoma, may not cause noticeable symptoms until significant damage has been done. Dilated eye exams should be performed around every two years or more often if directed by an eye doctor. Eye exams are essential for the early detection of eye disorders. Early diagnosis and treatment of eye disorders greatly improve the likelihood of preserving vision. Individuals with a family history of eye disorders or those with underlying medical conditions such as diabetes should be particularly diligent about regular eye appointments. Eye exams can detect issues that may be indicative of other health problems as well.

## CONCLUSION: EYE HEALTH FOR A LIFETIME OF CLEAR VISION

Maintaining good eye health is an ongoing process that requires attention and care. Adopting healthy lifestyle habits, such as good nutrition and regular physical activity, as well as regular eye exams and screenings, can go a long way in preventing eye disorders or managing them more effectively. Remember, good vision is essential for a life well-lived, so prioritize eye health to maintain a lifetime of clear vision.

## SUBCHAPTER 5.1: HEALTHY LIFESTYLE HABITS

Maintaining a healthy lifestyle is crucial for ensuring good eye health. Here are some healthy lifestyle habits to keep in mind:

## Eating a Healthy Diet

A healthy diet consisting of a variety of fruits and vegetables can provide essential vitamins, minerals, and antioxidants necessary for maintaining good eye health. Leafy greens, berries, and foods high in vitamin A, C, and E can help prevent eye diseases.

## Staying Hydrated

Drinking plenty of water can prevent dehydration and keep the eyes hydrated, reducing dry eye symptoms.

## Avoiding Smoking

Smoking significantly increases the risk of developing age-related macular degeneration, cataracts, and other eye diseases. Quitting smoking can decrease the risk of such eye disorders and improve overall health.

## Taking Breaks from Technology

Spending extended periods of time in front of a computer or phone screen can cause eye strain, which may lead to headaches, blurred vision, or dry eyes. Taking frequent breaks by looking away from the screen every 20 minutes and blinking regularly can help reduce eye strain.

# Wearing Sun Protection

Protecting the eyes from the harmful UV rays of the sun can prevent the development of cataracts, macular degeneration, and other eye disorders. Wearing wide-brimmed hats and sunglasses with UV protection when outdoors can help protect the eyes from harmful ultraviolet rays. By incorporating these healthy lifestyle habits into daily routines, individuals can protect their eyes from disease and maintain good eye health for a lifetime of clear vision.

## EYE EXAMS AND SCREENINGS

Regular eye exams and screenings are essential for maintaining good eye health. Eye exams are routine procedures that can help detect any issues with the eyes before they progress. Even if you do not wear glasses or contacts, you should still have your eyes checked regularly. An eye exam typically involves a series of tests that measure the sharpness of a person's vision, eye pressure, eye movement, and overall eye health. During the exam, the optometrist or ophthalmologist may also dilate your pupils to allow a more detailed examination of the retina and optic nerve. It is recommended that adults have a comprehensive eye exam at least once every two years. However, those with certain health conditions such as diabetes or high blood pressure may need more frequent eye exams. Children should also have their eyes examined regularly, as undiagnosed vision problems can negatively affect their academic performance. Eye screenings are quick assessments that can be performed by a school nurse or other healthcare professionals. Screening is generally done to identify any potential vision problems that may require further testing. Children should undergo vision screenings regularly to ensure their eyes are developing normally. The earlier eye issues are detected, the easier and more successful the treatment can be. Regular eye exams and screenings can help to prevent or minimize the impact of vision problems, allowing you to maintain clear vision and overall eye health for years to come. By scheduling routine eye exams and screenings, you are making an investment in your future eye health. Don't neglect your eyes, make an appointment with your eye care provider today!